DCRATES

Questions to Ask Your Doctor

Leslie Collins Cole, M.D.

Docrates: Questions to Ask Your Doctor
Copyright © 2013 Leslie Collins Cole. All rights reserved.

Cover Design:	Rita Frizzell/Marc Whitaker
Typesetting:	PerfecType, Nashville, TN
First printing:	2013
Website:	YourDocrates.com

ISBN: 978-1492829959

Printed by Amazon CreateSpace

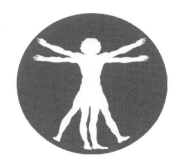

Contents

Introduction 5

My Medical History 8

Medications I Take 10

Vaccinations 16

Allergies to Medicines 17

My Medical Appointment 18

Upcoming Appointments. 94

My List of Doctors 98

Acknowledgments 101

Websites and Resources 102

Introduction

At my fortieth birthday dinner, as I was forking cake into my mouth, my mother casually said to her three children, "Oh, by the way, I had a biopsy of my breast and they want me to come back because they found something."

"What?! What did they find?"

"I can't remember."

"Did you write it down?"

"No."

"When do you go back?"

"I can't remember. Next week, I think."

How can she not remember this? I was frustrated and decided to go with her and speak to the doctor myself. I jotted a few questions on a little yellow piece of scrap paper. At her visit, when the doctor and resident walked into the clinic, my parents and I were suddenly like timid mice. Sitting on the patient side of the white coat, I began to sweat. My heart was beating too fast. My mother sat like a compliant little girl on the exam table in her paper gown, bare feet dangling, trying to appear strong. I asked my scribbled questions; the doctor answered. But in my trembling, I forgot to record his responses. By the afternoon, I was second-guessing what he had told me: *Was it HER2-receptor positive or negative?* I had lost the little scribbled paper. None of us remembered when mom was to have surgery, if she would need chemo, whom she was to call.

Answers are not answers unless they are preceded by questions.

One particular medical journal essay I read in my medical school years made a lasting impression on me: the article described the difference between Eastern education and Western education. In the East, the author wrote, the student's mind is prepared with questions before being given answers, like lining a closet with hooks (questions) onto which the answers could be hung. Prepare the mind with the question first; then search for the answer. Otherwise, the new information is not really an *answer*. In contrast, Western education conveys an onslaught of facts and information, and the learner is left to scramble to make those facts meaningful. I was living this second reality as a medical student: thousands and thousands of facts to memorize and categorize. We medical students even paid one student per class to record the daily onslaught of facts so as not to miss a single one of them. I swallowed this information like Lucille Ball choking down chocolates in the classic *I Love Lucy* episode!

Patients do not always have hooks—the questions—for the answers we doctors give them. And doctors may not always provide answers for the questions the patient is really asking. I found that some of my patients brought their own questions on little scraps of paper. Only a very few brought a pen and recorded answers.

You are not going to remember your answers unless you take notes.

Many of my patients were not remembering what we were discussing even a day later. If I could not remember my medical class facts without someone recording them for me, how would my patients remember what I was telling them if they weren't recording it? "What did she tell me I had? What test am I having?"

You want your doctor to understand you.

Many times patients come to the doctor visit with fear, embarrassment, or a desire not to be a bother to the doctor. The patient may be afraid to ask, *Is this cancer?* If the question the patient is most afraid to ask is understood and answered, the patient can feel that she has had a successful patient-doctor visit. To be understood is to be loved. I believe one reason people are moving towards holistic medicine is the desire to be heard, understood, and cared for. The lack of a sense of being understood drives unnecessary testing, doctor shopping, and unwarranted malpractice suits. Both parties must be prepared to have good communication. So, how can patients prepare for the conversation with the doctor?

Ask it. Remember it.

After that birthday dinner with my mother, the idea for *Docrates* came to me: a simple journal to organize the most important questions and answers from each doctor's visit. A resource to reassure the patient that it is good to ask, to be answered, and to be understood.

I drew my inspiration from Socrates, a Greek philosopher known for his method of inquiry and discussion between individuals, based on asking and answering questions to stimulate critical thinking and to illuminate ideas. Doctor + Socrates = *Docrates.*

Use *Docrates* at your doctor visits to ask questions and remember answers. Give *Docrates* to your father, aunt, grandmother, or husband to take to their appointments when you cannot go with them. Give it to your mother so that she will write down what type of breast cancer she has. By the way, my mother is a survivor of breast cancer.

If you have suggestions for making this a more helpful resource, I welcome your thoughts at YourDocrates.com!

Leslie Collins Cole, M.D.

My Medical History

List all conditions, illnesses, diseases:
(i.e., diabetes, anxiety, heart problems . . .)

**List any hospitalizations, surgeries, tests, or procedures:
(Where, when, for what . . .)**

Medications I Take

Pharmacy # _____

Medicine: _____

Doctor: _____

Date prescribed: _____

Dosage: _____

Continue: _____ Yes _____ No

Medicine: _____

Doctor: _____

Date prescribed: _____

Dosage: _____

Continue: _____ Yes _____ No

Medicine: _____

Doctor: _____

Date prescribed: _____

Dosage: _____

Continue: _____ Yes _____ No

Medicine: _____

Doctor: _____

Date prescribed: _____

Dosage: _____

Continue: _____ Yes _____ No

Medicine: _____

Doctor: _____

Date prescribed: _____

Dosage: _____

Continue: _____ Yes _____ No

Medicine: _____

Doctor: _____

Date prescribed: _____

Dosage: _____

Continue: _____ Yes _____ No

Medications I Take

Pharmacy # _____

Medicine: _____

Doctor: _____

Date prescribed: _____

Dosage: _____

Continue: _____ Yes _____ No

Medicine: _____

Doctor: _____

Date prescribed: _____

Dosage: _____

Continue: _____ Yes _____ No

Medicine: _____

Doctor: _____

Date prescribed: _____

Dosage: _____

Continue: _____ Yes _____ No

Medicine: _____

Doctor: _____

Date prescribed: _____

Dosage: _____

Continue: _____ Yes _____ No

Medicine: _____

Doctor: _____

Date prescribed: _____

Dosage: _____

Continue: _____ Yes _____ No

Medicine: _____

Doctor: _____

Date prescribed: _____

Dosage: _____

Continue: _____ Yes _____ No

Medications I Take

Pharmacy # _____

Medicine: _____

Doctor: _____

Date prescribed: _____

Dosage: _____

Continue: _____ Yes _____ No

Medicine: _____

Doctor: _____

Date prescribed: _____

Dosage: _____

Continue: _____ Yes _____ No

Medicine: _____

Doctor: _____

Date prescribed: _____

Dosage: _____

Continue: _____ Yes _____ No

Medicine:

Doctor:

Date prescribed:

Dosage:

Continue: _____ Yes _____ No

Medicine:

Doctor:

Date prescribed:

Dosage:

Continue: _____ Yes _____ No

Medicine:

Doctor:

Date prescribed:

Dosage:

Continue: _____ Yes _____ No

Vaccinations

What: _____

Date: _____

What: _____

Date: _____

What: _____

Date: _____

What: _____

Date: _____

What: _____

Date: _____

What: _____

Date: _____

What: _____

Date: _____

What: _____

Date: _____

Allergies to Medicines

Medicine: _____

Reaction: _____

Medicine: _____

Reaction: _____

Medicine: _____

Reaction: _____

Medicine: _____

Reaction: _____

Medicine: _____

Reaction: _____

Medicine: _____

Reaction: _____

Medicine: _____

Reaction: _____

Medicine: _____

Reaction: _____

My Medical Appointment

Doctor

Clinic Address

Clinic Phone #

Date

What to Mention to the Doctor

These are my most concerning symptoms:

1.

2.

3.

4.

5.

Questions to ask the doctor

What is my diagnosis/condition?

1.

2.

3.

What does my diagnosis mean?

Will I take medicines? What are their names and dosages?

Will I have tests?

What?

When?

Where?

How will I be notified of the results?

Test Results

If I need to call about a question, to whom will I speak?

What is the phone number I should use?

What question will I regret not having asked?

What question do I most want the doctor to understand?

Post-Appointment Thoughts

My Medical Appointment

Doctor

Clinic Address

Clinic Phone #

Date

What to Mention to the Doctor

These are my most concerning symptoms:

1.

2.

3.

4.

5.

Questions to ask the doctor

What is my diagnosis/condition?

1.

2.

3.

What does my diagnosis mean?

My Medical Appointment (continued)

Will I take medicines? What are their names and dosages?

Will I have tests?

What?

When?

Where?

How will I be notified of the results?

Test Results

If I need to call about a question, to whom will I speak?

What is the phone number I should use?

What question will I regret not having asked?

What question do I most want the doctor to understand?

Post-Appointment Thoughts

My Medical Appointment

Doctor

Clinic Address

Clinic Phone #

Date

What to Mention to the Doctor

These are my most concerning symptoms:

1.

2.

3.

4.

5.

Questions to ask the doctor

What is my diagnosis/condition?

1. _____

_____

_____

2. _____

_____

_____

3. _____

_____

_____

What does my diagnosis mean?

_____

_____

_____

_____

_____

_____

_____

_____

_____

_____

My Medical Appointment (continued)

Will I take medicines? What are their names and dosages?

Will I have tests?

What?

When?

Where?

How will I be notified of the results?

Test Results

If I need to call about a question, to whom will I speak?

What is the phone number I should use?

What question will I regret not having asked?

What question do I most want the doctor to understand?

Post-Appointment Thoughts

My Medical Appointment

Doctor

Clinic Address

Clinic Phone #

Date

What to Mention to the Doctor

These are my most concerning symptoms:

1.

2.

3.

4.

5.

Questions to ask the doctor

What is my diagnosis/condition?

1. _____

_____

_____

2. _____

_____

_____

3. _____

_____

_____

What does my diagnosis mean?

_____

_____

_____

_____

_____

_____

_____

_____

_____

_____

My Medical Appointment (continued)

Will I take medicines? What are their names and dosages?

Will I have tests?

What? _____

When? _____

Where? _____

How will I be notified of the results?

Test Results

If I need to call about a question, to whom will I speak?

What is the phone number I should use?

What question will I regret not having asked?

What question do I most want the doctor to understand?

Post-Appointment Thoughts

My Medical Appointment

Doctor

Clinic Address

Clinic Phone #

Date

What to Mention to the Doctor

These are my most concerning symptoms:

1.

2.

3.

4.

5.

Questions to ask the doctor

What is my diagnosis/condition?

1. _____

_____

_____

2. _____

_____

_____

3. _____

_____

_____

What does my diagnosis mean?

_____

_____

_____

_____

_____

_____

_____

_____

_____

_____

My Medical Appointment (continued)

Will I take medicines? What are their names and dosages?

Will I have tests?

What?

When?

Where?

How will I be notified of the results?

Test Results

If I need to call about a question, to whom will I speak?

What is the phone number I should use?

What question will I regret not having asked?

What question do I most want the doctor to understand?

Post-Appointment Thoughts

My Medical Appointment

Doctor

Clinic Address

Clinic Phone #

Date

What to Mention to the Doctor

These are my most concerning symptoms:

1.

2.

3.

4.

5.

Questions to ask the doctor

What is my diagnosis/condition?

1. _____

_____

_____

2. _____

_____

_____

3. _____

_____

_____

What does my diagnosis mean?

_____

_____

_____

_____

_____

_____

_____

_____

_____

_____

Will I take medicines? What are their names and dosages?

Will I have tests?

What? _____

When? _____

Where?_____

How will I be notified of the results?

Test Results

If I need to call about a question, to whom will I speak?

What is the phone number I should use?

What question will I regret not having asked?

What question do I most want the doctor to understand?

Post-Appointment Thoughts

My Medical Appointment

Doctor

Clinic Address

Clinic Phone #

Date

What to Mention to the Doctor

These are my most concerning symptoms:

1.

2.

3.

4.

5.

Questions to ask the doctor

What is my diagnosis/condition?

1. _____

_____

_____

2. _____

_____

_____

3. _____

_____

_____

What does my diagnosis mean?

_____

_____

_____

_____

_____

_____

_____

_____

_____

_____

Will I take medicines? What are their names and dosages?

Will I have tests?

What?

When?

Where?

How will I be notified of the results?

Test Results

If I need to call about a question, to whom will I speak?

What is the phone number I should use?

What question will I regret not having asked?

What question do I most want the doctor to understand?

Post-Appointment Thoughts

My Medical Appointment

Doctor

Clinic Address

Clinic Phone #

Date

What to Mention to the Doctor

These are my most concerning symptoms:

1.

2.

3.

4.

5.

Questions to ask the doctor

What is my diagnosis/condition?

1.

2.

3.

What does my diagnosis mean?

My Medical Appointment (continued)

Will I take medicines? What are their names and dosages?

Will I have tests?

What?

When?

Where?

How will I be notified of the results?

Test Results

If I need to call about a question, to whom will I speak?

What is the phone number I should use?

What question will I regret not having asked?

What question do I most want the doctor to understand?

Post-Appointment Thoughts

My Medical Appointment

Doctor

Clinic Address

Clinic Phone #

Date

What to Mention to the Doctor

These are my most concerning symptoms:

1.

2.

3.

4.

5.

Questions to ask the doctor

What is my diagnosis/condition?

1. _____

_____

_____

2. _____

_____

_____

3. _____

_____

_____

What does my diagnosis mean?

_____

_____

_____

_____

_____

_____

_____

_____

_____

_____

Will I take medicines? What are their names and dosages?

Will I have tests?

What?

When?

Where?

How will I be notified of the results?

Test Results

If I need to call about a question, to whom will I speak?

What is the phone number I should use?

What question will I regret not having asked?

What question do I most want the doctor to understand?

Post-Appointment Thoughts

My Medical Appointment

Doctor _____

Clinic Address _____

Clinic Phone # _____

Date _____

What to Mention to the Doctor

These are my most concerning symptoms:

1. _____

_____

_____

2. _____

_____

_____

3. _____

_____

_____

4. _____

_____

_____

5. _____

_____

_____

Questions to ask the doctor

What is my diagnosis/condition?

1.

2.

3.

What does my diagnosis mean?

Will I take medicines? What are their names and dosages?

Will I have tests?

What?

When?

Where?

How will I be notified of the results?

Test Results

If I need to call about a question, to whom will I speak?

What is the phone number I should use?

What question will I regret not having asked?

What question do I most want the doctor to understand?

Post-Appointment Thoughts

My Medical Appointment

Doctor _____

Clinic Address _____

Clinic Phone # _____

Date _____

What to Mention to the Doctor

These are my most concerning symptoms:

1. _____

_____

_____

2. _____

_____

_____

3. _____

_____

_____

4. _____

_____

_____

5. _____

_____

_____

Questions to ask the doctor

What is my diagnosis/condition?

1.

2.

3.

What does my diagnosis mean?

My Medical Appointment (continued)

Will I take medicines? What are their names and dosages?

Will I have tests?

What?

When?

Where?

How will I be notified of the results?

Test Results

If I need to call about a question, to whom will I speak?

What is the phone number I should use?

What question will I regret not having asked?

What question do I most want the doctor to understand?

Post-Appointment Thoughts

My Medical Appointment

Doctor _____

Clinic Address _____

Clinic Phone # _____

Date _____

What to Mention to the Doctor

These are my most concerning symptoms:

1. _____

_____

_____

2. _____

_____

_____

3. _____

_____

_____

4. _____

_____

_____

5. _____

_____

_____

Questions to ask the doctor

What is my diagnosis/condition?

1. _____

_____

_____

2. _____

_____

_____

3. _____

_____

_____

What does my diagnosis mean?

_____

_____

_____

_____

_____

_____

_____

_____

_____

Will I take medicines? What are their names and dosages?

Will I have tests?

What? _____

When? _____

Where? _____

How will I be notified of the results?

Test Results

If I need to call about a question, to whom will I speak?

What is the phone number I should use?

What question will I regret not having asked?

What question do I most want the doctor to understand?

Post-Appointment Thoughts

My Medical Appointment

Doctor ....

Clinic Address ....

Clinic Phone # ....

Date ....

What to Mention to the Doctor

These are my most concerning symptoms:

1. ....

....

....

2. ....

....

....

3. ....

....

....

4. ....

....

....

5. ....

....

....

Questions to ask the doctor

What is my diagnosis/condition?

1.

2.

3.

What does my diagnosis mean?

Will I take medicines? What are their names and dosages?

Will I have tests?

What?

When?

Where?

How will I be notified of the results?

Test Results

If I need to call about a question, to whom will I speak?

What is the phone number I should use?

What question will I regret not having asked?

What question do I most want the doctor to understand?

Post-Appointment Thoughts

My Medical Appointment

Doctor

Clinic Address

Clinic Phone #

Date

What to Mention to the Doctor

These are my most concerning symptoms:

1.

2.

3.

4.

5.

Questions to ask the doctor

What is my diagnosis/condition?

1.

2.

3.

What does my diagnosis mean?

Will I take medicines? What are their names and dosages?

_____

_____

_____

_____

Will I have tests?

What? _____

When? _____

Where? _____

How will I be notified of the results?

_____

_____

Test Results

_____

_____

_____

_____

_____

_____

If I need to call about a question, to whom will I speak?

What is the phone number I should use?

What question will I regret not having asked?

What question do I most want the doctor to understand?

Post-Appointment Thoughts

My Medical Appointment

Doctor _____

Clinic Address _____

Clinic Phone # _____

Date _____

What to Mention to the Doctor

These are my most concerning symptoms:

1. _____

   _____

   _____

2. _____

   _____

   _____

3. _____

   _____

   _____

4. _____

   _____

   _____

5. _____

   _____

   _____

Questions to ask the doctor

What is my diagnosis/condition?

1.

2.

3.

What does my diagnosis mean?

Will I take medicines? What are their names and dosages?

Will I have tests?

What? _____

When? _____

Where? _____

How will I be notified of the results?

Test Results

If I need to call about a question, to whom will I speak?

What is the phone number I should use?

What question will I regret not having asked?

What question do I most want the doctor to understand?

Post-Appointment Thoughts

My Medical Appointment

Doctor _____

Clinic Address _____

Clinic Phone # _____

Date _____

What to Mention to the Doctor

These are my most concerning symptoms:

1. _____
_____
_____

2. _____
_____
_____

3. _____
_____
_____

4. _____
_____
_____

5. _____
_____
_____

Questions to ask the doctor

What is my diagnosis/condition?

1.

2.

3.

What does my diagnosis mean?

My Medical Appointment (continued)

Will I take medicines? What are their names and dosages?

Will I have tests?

What?

When?

Where?

How will I be notified of the results?

Test Results

If I need to call about a question, to whom will I speak?

What is the phone number I should use?

What question will I regret not having asked?

What question do I most want the doctor to understand?

Post-Appointment Thoughts

My Medical Appointment

Doctor _____

Clinic Address _____

Clinic Phone # _____

Date _____

What to Mention to the Doctor

These are my most concerning symptoms:

1. _____

    _____

    _____

2. _____

    _____

    _____

3. _____

    _____

    _____

4. _____

    _____

    _____

5. _____

    _____

    _____

Questions to ask the doctor

What is my diagnosis/condition?

1.

2.

3.

What does my diagnosis mean?

Will I take medicines? What are their names and dosages?

Will I have tests?

What?

When?

Where?

How will I be notified of the results?

Test Results

If I need to call about a question, to whom will I speak?

What is the phone number I should use?

What question will I regret not having asked?

What question do I most want the doctor to understand?

Post-Appointment Thoughts

My Medical Appointment

Doctor _____

Clinic Address _____

Clinic Phone # _____

Date _____

What to Mention to the Doctor

These are my most concerning symptoms:

1. _____

_____

_____

2. _____

_____

_____

3. _____

_____

_____

4. _____

_____

_____

5. _____

_____

_____

Questions to ask the doctor

What is my diagnosis/condition?

1.

2.

3.

What does my diagnosis mean?

My Medical Appointment (continued)

Will I take medicines? What are their names and dosages?

Will I have tests?

What?

When?

Where?

How will I be notified of the results?

Test Results

If I need to call about a question, to whom will I speak?

What is the phone number I should use?

What question will I regret not having asked?

What question do I most want the doctor to understand?

Post-Appointment Thoughts

My Medical Appointment

Doctor _____

Clinic Address _____

Clinic Phone # _____

Date _____

What to Mention to the Doctor

These are my most concerning symptoms:

1. _____
   _____
   _____

2. _____
   _____
   _____

3. _____
   _____
   _____

4. _____
   _____
   _____

5. _____
   _____
   _____

Questions to ask the doctor

What is my diagnosis/condition?

1. _____

2. _____

3. _____

What does my diagnosis mean?

Will I take medicines? What are their names and dosages?

Will I have tests?

What?

When?

Where?

How will I be notified of the results?

Test Results

If I need to call about a question, to whom will I speak?

What is the phone number I should use?

What question will I regret not having asked?

What question do I most want the doctor to understand?

Post-Appointment Thoughts

Upcoming Appointments

My List of Doctors

Use this list to record information about all your doctors, specialists, dentists, therapists, chiropractors, etc.

Name _____ Specialty _____

Phone _____ FAX _____

Name _____ Specialty _____

Phone _____ FAX _____

Name _____ Specialty _____

Phone _____ FAX _____

Name _____ Specialty _____

Phone _____ FAX _____

Name _____ Specialty _____

Phone _____ FAX _____

Name _____ Specialty _____

Phone _____ FAX _____

Name _____ Specialty _____

Phone _____ FAX _____

Name _____ Specialty _____

Phone _____ FAX _____

Name _____ Specialty _____

Phone _____ FAX _____

Name _____ Specialty _____

Phone _____ FAX _____

Name _____ Specialty _____

Phone _____ FAX _____

Name _____ Specialty _____

Phone _____ FAX _____

Name _____ Specialty _____

Phone _____ FAX _____

Name _____ Specialty _____

Phone _____ FAX _____

Acknowledgments

To these people, I express my gratitude:

- My family and friends for their encouragement, prayer, great ideas, and support.
- My *The Artist's Way* group for encouragement, great ideas, and laughter.
- Robin Pippin, who has met and brainstormed with me, sent lots of email, and encouraged and edited this tool book. She also introduced me to these people to whom I'm grateful:
- Graphic designers Rita Frizzell and Marc Whitaker; Kristin Goble of PerfecType; and Janice Neely, the marketing and networking guru. Thank you all for distilling this idea into a real thing.
- Tim, my husband, for your love, humor, and best-friendedness, without which this book would not have happened.

At 19, I learned that Bach and several famous composers had inscribed "S.D.G" at the end of their compositions: *Soli Deo Gloria.* I admired and envied this declaration. The idea for this book landed on me like an answer. So I, too, write **S.D.G.**

Websites and Resources

Made in the USA
San Bernardino, CA
20 February 2014